FOOD AND HYGIENE

First published in the United States in 1990 by
Gloucester Press, 387 Park Avenue South, New York, NY 10016

Design: Andy Wilkinson, Rob Hillier
Editor: Catherine Bradley
Picture research: Cecilia Weston-Baker
Illustrator: Ron Hayward Associates
Consultant: Angela Grunsell

The publishers would like to acknowledge that the photographs reproduced in this book have been posed by models or have been obtained from photographic agencies.

Library of Congress Cataloging-in-Publication Data
Sanders, Pete.
    Food and hygiene / Pete Sanders.
        p. cm. -- (Let's talk about)
    Summary: Examines the many questions children ask about food, from additives to pesticides, from fast foods to vitamin pills. Encourages children to think about what they are eating and what is the best way to feed themselves.
    ISBN 0-531-17243-0
    1. Nutrition--Juvenile literature. [1. Nutrition.] I. Title.
RA784.S339 1990
613.2--dc20
                                            90-3246 CIP AC

"LET'S TALK ABOUT"

FOOD AND HYGIENE

PETE SANDERS

Gloucester Press
London · New York · Toronto · Sydney

"Why do we eat the food that we do?"

We all have our favorite foods. Some people like savory tastes, others have a sweet tooth. Most children don't choose or prepare their own food. Adults do this for them. Every country and many regions have special foods. Some people find it hard to try foods that are not familiar to them. Some meals can remind us of Christmas or Thanksgiving. Sometimes we go along with what other people like to eat. Some people eat for comfort. Have you ever eaten just because you were bored? Others lead busy lives and make do with convenience food or go to fast-food restaurants.

This book will help you understand the reasons behind choosing food. It will also tell you about what to remember when choosing, preparing and eating food.

How food looks can be as important as its texture and taste.

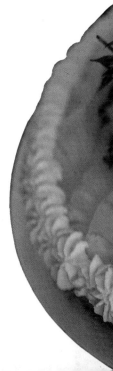

4

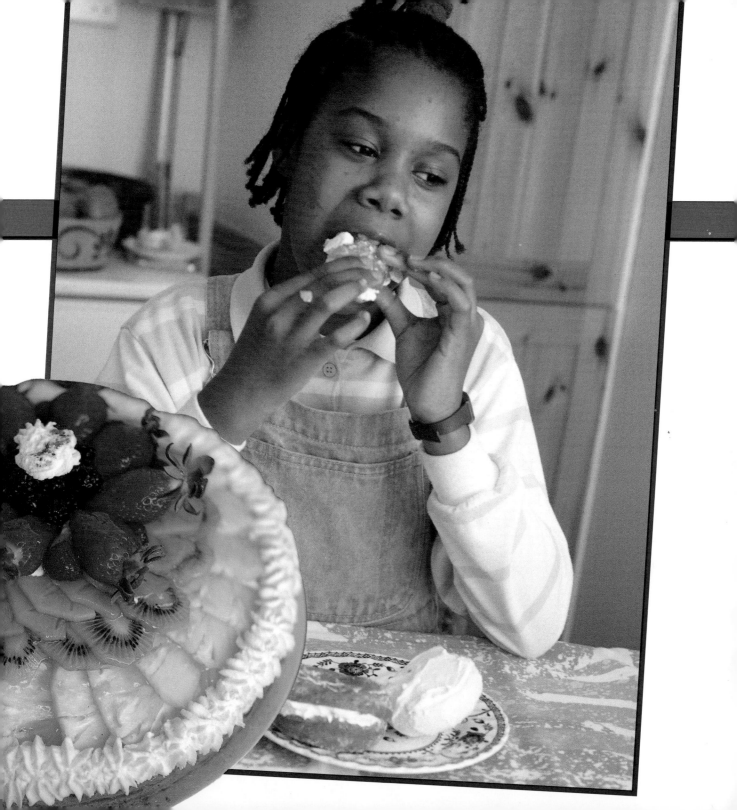

"Why can't I just eat what I want?"

There are all kinds of food you can eat. Yet everyone has their favorites. Some of you may not see anything wrong in eating what you like. But food is more than just eating something you like. You have to think about what you eat, when you eat it, and what it will do for you. Eating different kinds of foods keeps you healthy and strong.

Sometimes you can't eat what you want because it is too expensive. Some foods, like strawberries, may not be available all year round. Others may be very expensive to produce, such as caviar. The food you eat at school might not be what you like. Often what you want to eat may depend on your mood. Some children would like to eat ice cream all day, but most families only allow children to eat it as a treat. Some people can become ill if they eat certain foods, or too much of the same food. It is not always possible for you to choose what to eat, because it is not you who buys the food.

Every country has its special foods. Chinese food is eaten in restaurants all over the world. This Chinese meal is a very healthy mixture of rice and vegetables, and a little meat, poultry or fish.

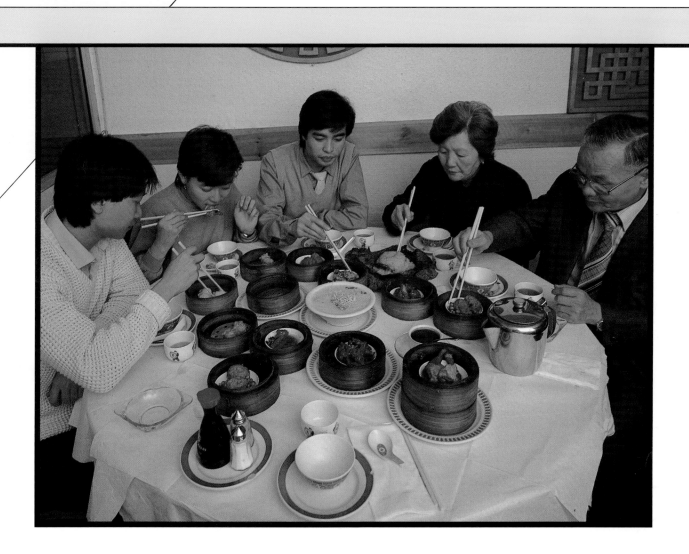

"Why do I need to eat different kinds of food?"

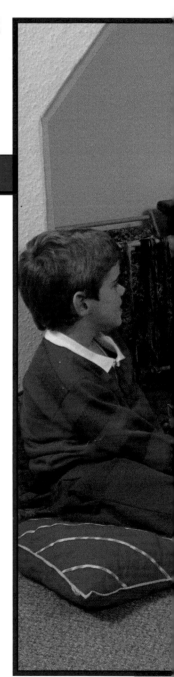

Just think of what you do during the day. You will be running around, playing, thinking and studying. At the same time your body is doing things which you may not have thought about. Have you thought about the ways that you are continually growing? Your body is made up of millions of tiny parts, called cells, which are being made all the time. Different cells do different things; for instance, cells in the blood protect us against illness. All of this takes a lot of energy. You get this energy from food. Food helps you to stay alive, to grow and be healthy. There is no one type of food that does this by itself. Different foods contain different nutrients, which make the body's cells work properly.

Even when you are doing something quietly, your body needs the energy it gets from food.

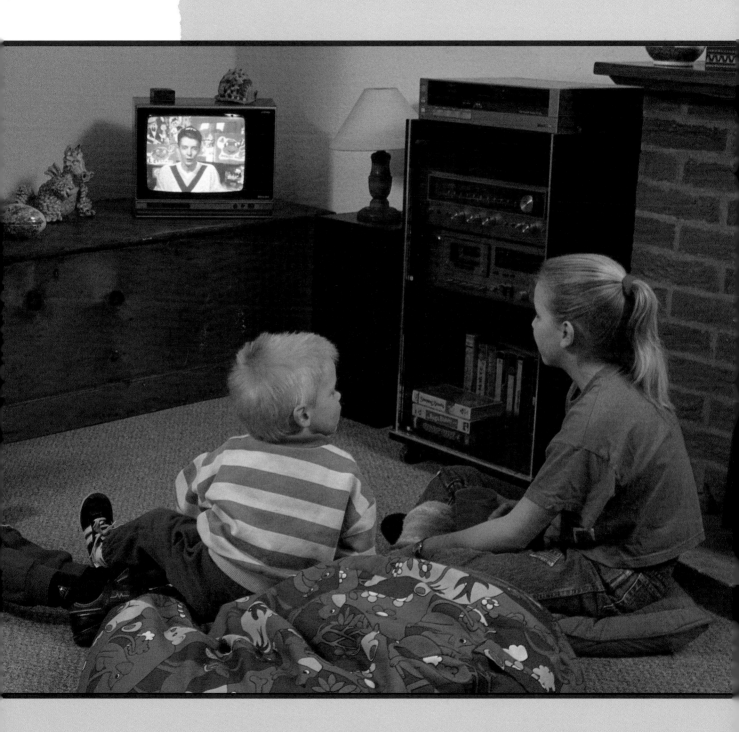

"What are nutrients?"

Nutrients in food help your body to grow properly and stay healthy. These nutrients are called protein, carbohydrates, fiber, fat, vitamins and minerals. Your body takes protein from meat, fish, milk, eggs, cheese, nuts, beans, peas and grains. Protein is used by your body to build cells. Carbohydrates give you energy. The main types of carbohydrates are starches and sugars. You get starches when you eat bread, potatoes, pasta, rice, flour and breakfast cereals. Sugar is found in different products. For example, tomato ketchup has a lot of sugar in it.

Another way we get energy is by eating fats. Butter, lard, vegetable oils, cream and milk contain a lot of fat. Fiber helps food move through the body. Beans and whole grains contain a lot of fiber. Vitamins and minerals help to fight illness. For example, Vitamin C helps prevent you from bruising easily, having bleeding gums or losing your hair.

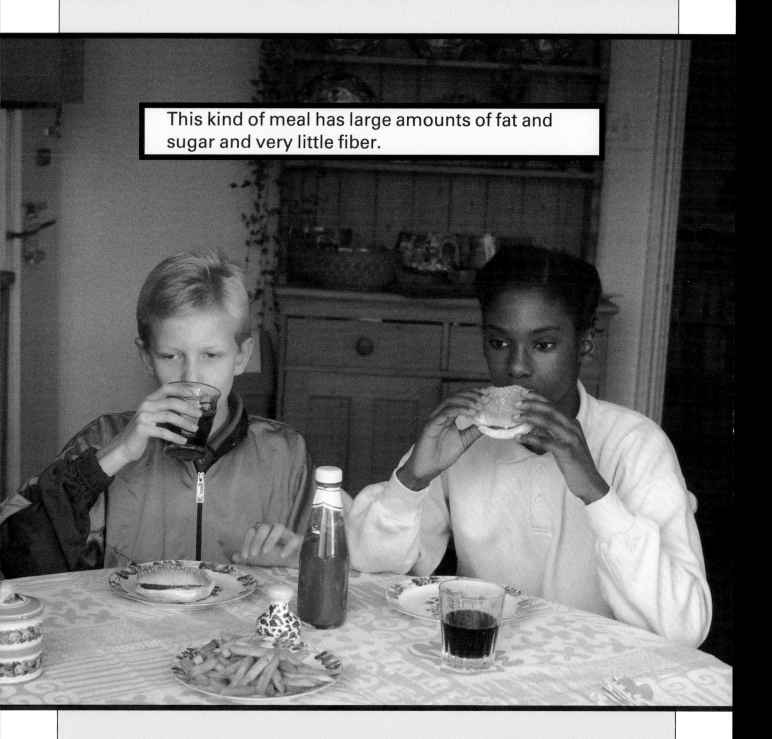

This kind of meal has large amounts of fat and sugar and very little fiber.

"What happens to food inside my body?"

Food cannot be used by the body until it has been changed in some way. This change is called digestion. You may know that food begins to change as you chew it in your mouth. Your teeth cut and grind it. Your mouth makes a juice called saliva, which makes food soft, so that you can swallow it. Your body squeezes the food through a tube to your stomach. There it is mixed with juices in your stomach. These change the food yet again.

Then the mixture of food and juices pass on into the small intestine. This also makes juices which mix with the food. The food is now a thin liquid and the nutrients can reach all the parts of the body through your bloodstream. Some of the food is left behind and passes into the large intestine. Here most of the water is taken out. At this stage, the food which is left behind in the large intestine is not needed by your body. You get rid of this when you go to the bathroom.

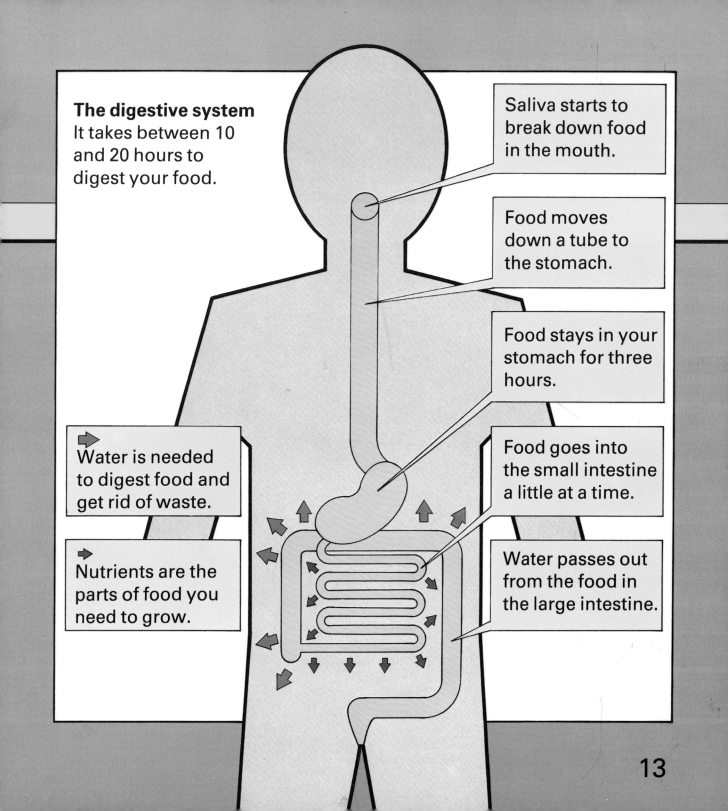

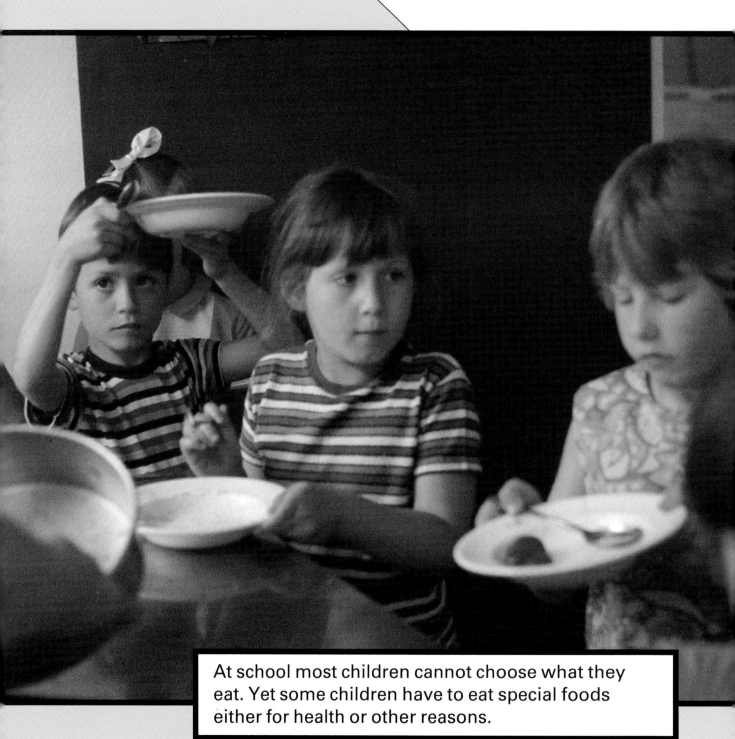

At school most children cannot choose what they eat. Yet some children have to eat special foods either for health or other reasons.

"Why do some people not eat certain foods?"

Some people cannot eat certain foods because of their health. For example, people with diabetes have to be very careful about how much sugar they eat. Those with heart problems are advised to eat less fat and salt. Others do not eat certain foods because of their religion. They may be vegetarian, or they may only eat certain meats.

Some people choose not to eat meat. They may not like the idea of eating an animal or be concerned about how animals are treated on farms. Many vegetarians feel that eating meat is an expensive way of feeding human beings. Others will not buy food that is produced in a country where the growers are treated unfairly. Some people will not buy fruits and vegetables that have been sprayed with chemicals. They believe these foods may damage their health. You may know someone who only eats certain foods because they are trying to lose weight.

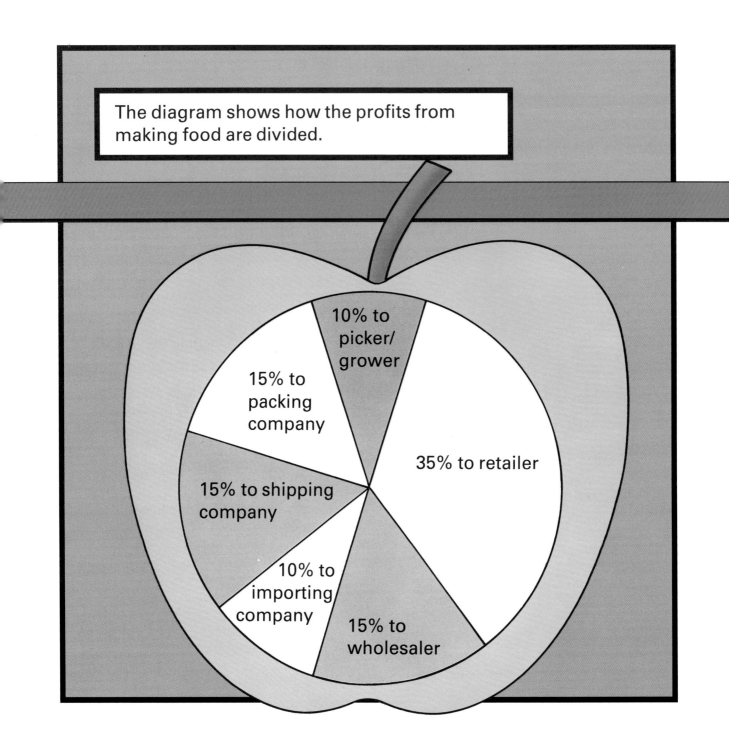

The diagram shows how the profits from making food are divided.

10% to picker/grower

15% to packing company

35% to retailer

15% to shipping company

10% to importing company

15% to wholesaler

"Why doesn't everybody have enough food?"

There is enough food produced in the world to feed everybody. But in every country some people go hungry. In Britain some people do not have enough money to buy the food that will keep them healthy. In poorer countries like Peru or India, there are people who are starving. The problem is that food is too expensive for them to buy. In some poor countries rich landowners or international companies control the land and use it to produce crops that are going to be sold elsewhere. Poor people cannot just grow their own food because they don't have any land.

Sometimes lack of rain or plagues of pests lead to local food shortages which can result in famines. In these cases other countries send in food aid, as well as seeds to plant next season's crops. Farmers in poorer countries need national and international help to be able to grow more food crops to feed their own people.

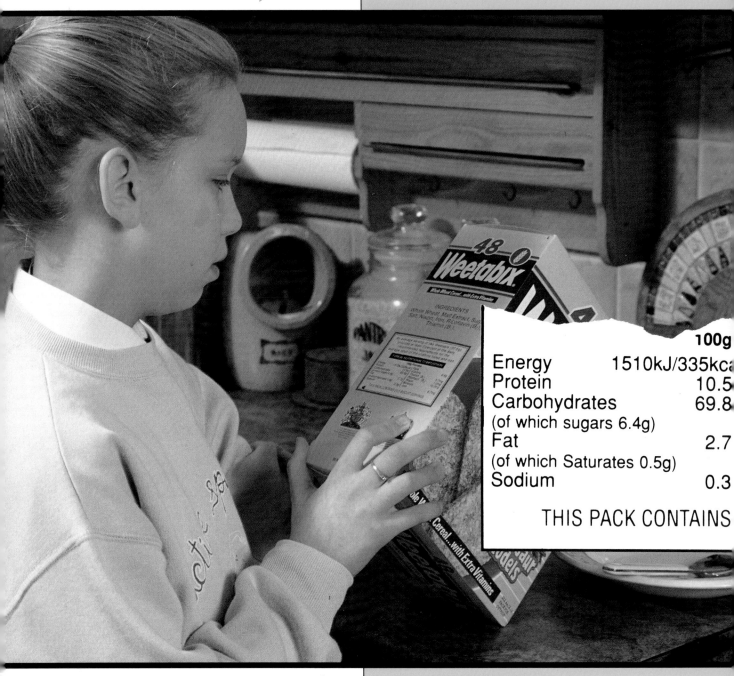

Whole Wheat, Malt

Niacin, Iron, Riboflav
Thiamin (B$_1$).

	100g
Energy	1510kJ/335kca
Protein	10.5
Carbohydrates	69.8
(of which sugars 6.4g)	
Fat	2.7
(of which Saturates 0.5g)	
Sodium	0.3

THIS PACK CONTAINS

48

Weetabix

"What happens to food before I eat it?"

Much of the food you eat is processed in some way. In the kitchen you will find canned food, dried foods, food in bottles and frozen foods. You know that if you leave food, it will go bad. People put food in the refrigerator to stop it from spoiling. Manufacturers use chemicals called preservatives to make the food last for a longer time. Some of these are specially made, others are natural. For example, salt is used to preserve some meats. Manufacturers also use colorings to give food the "right look." Flavor enhancers are used to give food a stronger flavor and emulsifiers are used to make food smooth.

9.4g

(B$_1$) 0.7mg
in (B$_2$) 1.0mg
10.0mg

6.7mg

IT SERVINGS

The ingredients on a label are listed in a certain order to show how much of each is in the food. There are no special preservatives in this food, but vitamins have been added.

Preservatives, colorings, flavor enhancers and emulsifiers are called additives. This means they have been added to food. Not everyone agrees that additives should be used in the preparation of food. Although it is said that they help to keep prices low and prevent food poisoning, some people think that they can lead to allergies and health problems. You can tell if food contains any additives by looking at the label, where they should be clearly marked.

Food can be prepared in lots of different ways. Even with food that you eat raw, such as fruit, you probably have been told that it is important to wash it first. After all, insecticides may have been used to grow the fruit and might still be on it. Some fruits and vegetables have to be peeled. Food that has been frozen sometimes needs to be defrosted before it can be cooked. Here it is very important to look at the instructions. Quite often labels will tell you how long to cook the food, and the way that this should be done.

Some people worry about microwave ovens. Not all ovens have the same power, and cooking times may need to be adjusted. It is easy to forget that having more than one item of food in the microwave makes a difference to how long it takes for things to cook. People are more and more aware of the importance of checking how well food is cooked.

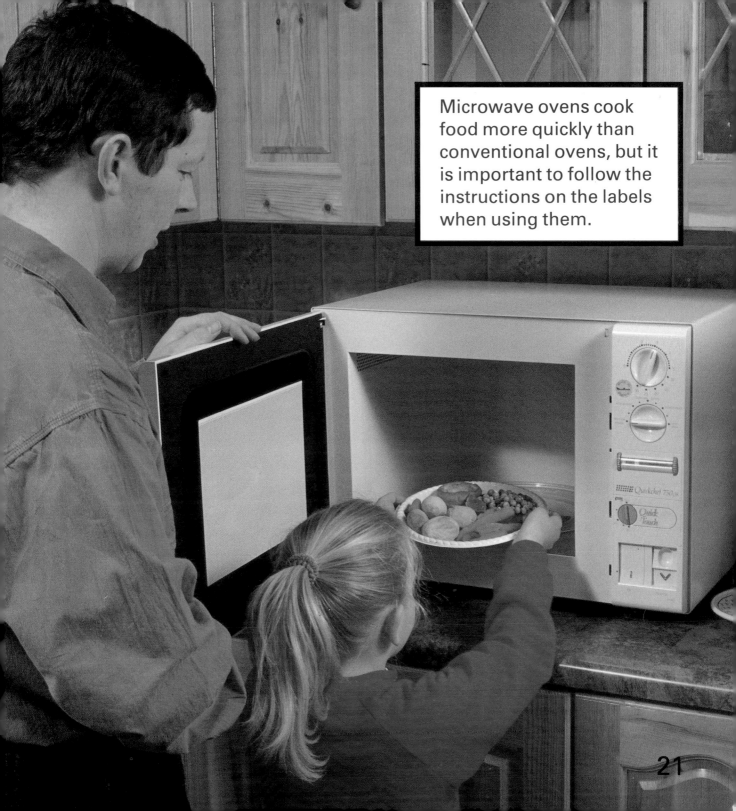

Microwave ovens cook food more quickly than conventional ovens, but it is important to follow the instructions on the labels when using them.

21

"Why are foods stored in different ways?"

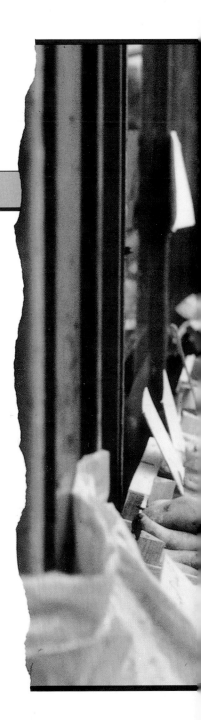

Foods are stored in boxes, in plastic, in paper, in cans, in jars and sometimes in foil. Packaging protects the food from dirt and bugs. Some foods are frozen to make them last longer than fresh ones. Canned food lasts even longer.

You have to be careful how you store food. Chilled and frozen foods need to be kept at a certain temperature. That is why it is important to put them straight into the refrigerator or freezer at home as soon as possible. If you don't, germs will breed as the temperature of the food changes. Foods can spoil if the refrigerator temperature is not set correctly. Raw meats should never come into contact with cooked or ready-to-eat food. Most stores display them in different places.

No matter how well food is stored, it will eventually go bad. Good shoppers look at the "sell by" or "best before" date. These dates are important because they say when the food is at its best.

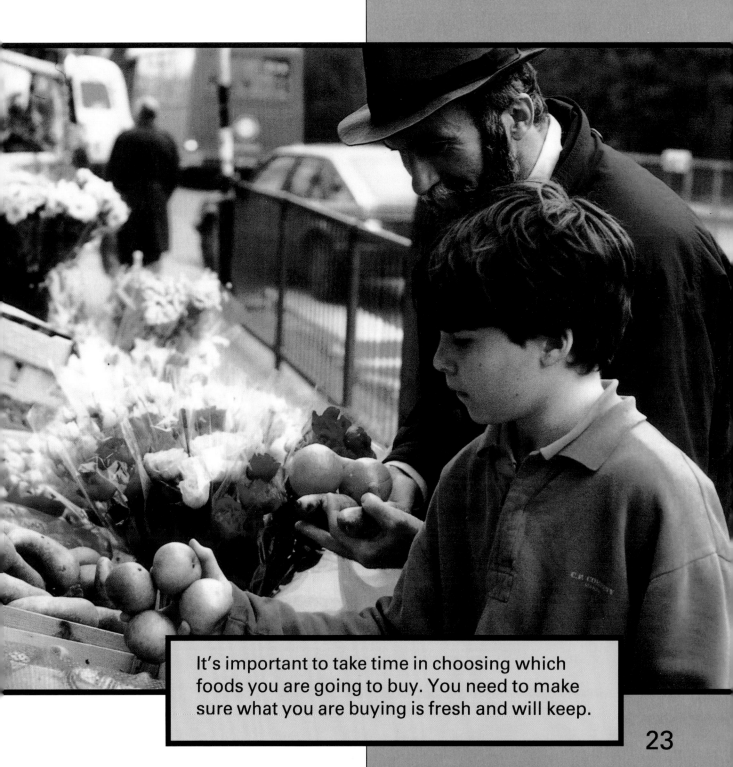

It's important to take time in choosing which foods you are going to buy. You need to make sure what you are buying is fresh and will keep.

23

"Why is it important to keep food clean?"

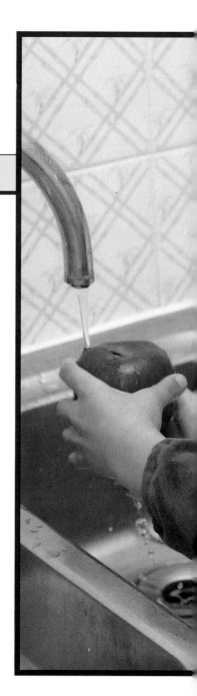

You will already know that it is important to store food in containers in the kitchen. Apart from getting rid of pesticides, washing food will get rid of some germs too. Germs can get into food at home. That is why kitchen surfaces, plates, cutlery, and pots and pans have to be kept clean. A small amount of food can become moldy and spread germs. Germs multiply in a warm kitchen. They get into cracked dishes, and even onto dishcloths and towels. The trouble with germs is that you cannot see them. You would need a microscope to see most germs. It seems easier when you actually see things that might make you ill. If you saw a caterpillar on a lettuce, you would wash it thoroughly.

People wash vegetables and fruit with care, because they know that many of them are sprayed with pesticides.

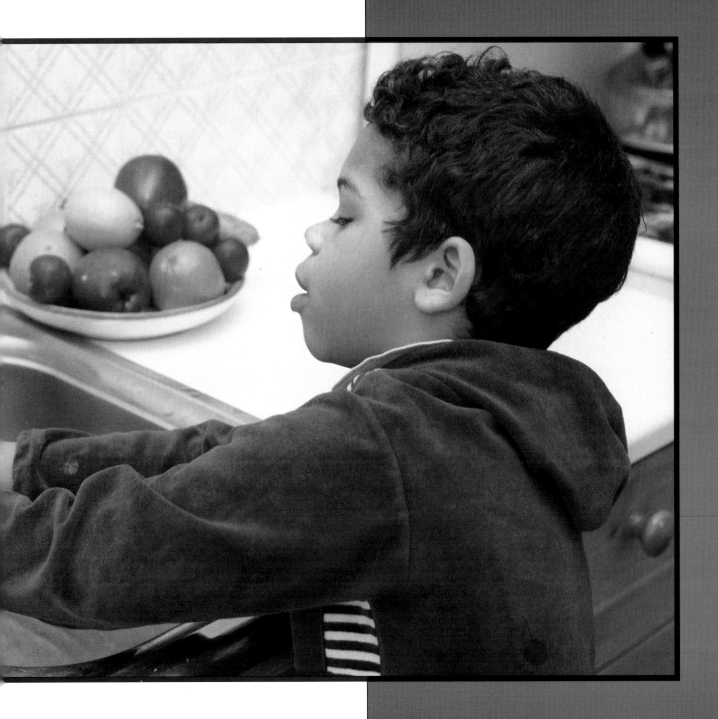

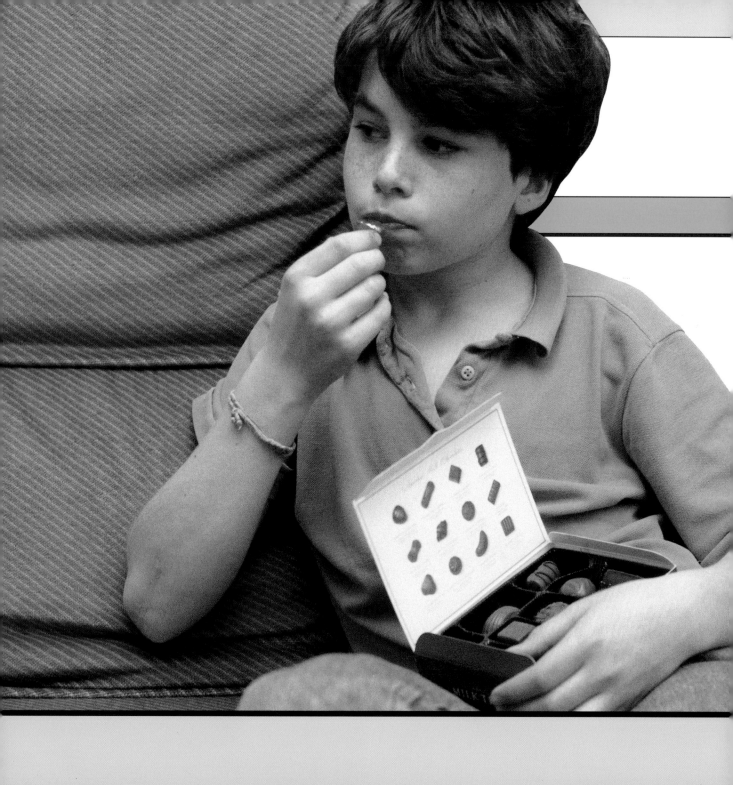

"Can some foods make me ill?"

Germs can easily grow inside food if it is not stored properly. You may have heard of listeria. These are the germs that breed when chilled food is not stored at the right temperature. Salmonella is another kind of germ that is killed during cooking. That is why it is important to cook certain foods, like eggs, chicken and turkey, very thoroughly to kill the salmonella.

Eating only one type of food can make you ill. For instance if people eat too many fats over a long time, the blood vessels leading from the heart may become blocked. Doctors advise people with heart problems to stop eating fats and salt.

There is a lot of sugar in chocolate, and this can harm your teeth. It is interesting that in some countries where people don't eat a lot of sugar, they have fewer problems with their teeth.

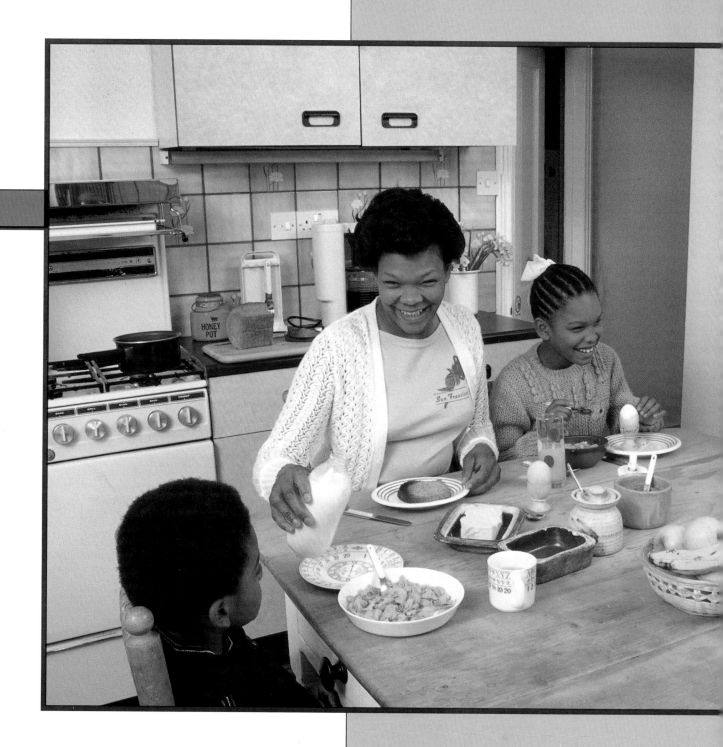

"What is healthy eating?"

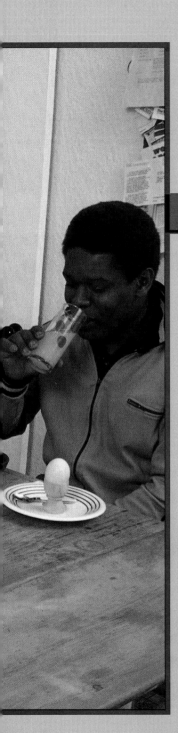

You may have heard about a "balanced diet." What this means is that we should eat a variety of foods, which will supply the body with all the nutrients it needs. Some adults have made decisions to eat less of some foods and more of others. They know that too much fat and sugar can make them unhealthy.

Healthy eating means eating cereals, bread, vegetables and fruits as well as milk, cheese, yogurt, lean meat, poultry, fish, nuts and eggs. It means not eating too much sugar, salt, butter, margarine and oil. Sugar gives you energy, but is bad for your teeth. Salt and fats can give you health problems in the future.

It is important to start the day with a good meal, which will give you energy for the things you need to do.

"What can I do?"

If you have read this book, you may have lots of ideas about what you might do. You realize that it is good to eat lots of cereal, vegetables and fruit. Because fried food is cooked in oils, you might want to try some foods grilled instead. Washing your hands before handling or eating food is also important as you may have some germs on them.

If you get hungry between meals, it is best not to have things that contain a lot of sugar. Eating too much sugar can lead to tooth decay. Also some people put on weight if they eat foods that contain lots of sugar. There are many different names for sugar, such as glucose, fructose and sucrose. Knowing them is helpful. Food manufacturers want us to buy what they make, so reading the ingredients will help you make sure that you are eating healthily.

You may find that many of the foods you eat are not chosen by you. It may be difficult to share ideas about a balanced diet, especially when it is not you who is paying for the food. Often adults can seem too busy to think about the food they eat. Those who are keeping an eye on what they eat sometimes keep a diary. In it they list the kinds of food they have. You might want to ask adults around you to help to plan your diary.

What the words mean?

carbohydrates food containing a lot of starch and sugar. They give you energy.

digestion the breaking down of food into tiny pieces so that it can be passed into the bloodstream.

fats foods that give you energy. They can feel very greasy, such as butter.

fiber the parts of fruits, vegetables and other plants that you eat, but which cannot be digested.

germs tiny living things which grow on food and make it decay and go bad. Some of them cause diseases.

minerals these are found in all kinds of food and keep you healthy. Calcium and iron are two kinds of minerals which you must have to stay healthy.

proteins foods which help you grow and repair damaged and worn-out parts of the body.

vitamins are often named after the letters of the alphabet. You need to eat a small amount of each vitamin to stay healthy.

Index